THE CELERY JUICE CLEANSE HACK: A 7 STEP GUIDE TO FLUSH TOXINS AND RESTORE LIVER HEALTH

Relief for Relief for Brain Fog, Acne, Eczema, ADHD, Thyroid Disorders, Diabetes, SIBO, Acid Reflux and Lyme Disease

GABRIELLE TOWNSEND

Silk Publishing

Introduction

If you don't take care of this the most magnificent machine that you will ever be given...where are you going to live?

— KARYN CALABRESE

Congratulations on purchasing *The Celery Juice Cleanse Hack,* and thank you for doing so. Are you ready to feel better and improve your mind, body, and spirit? If so, keep reading. What you choose to eat has a lifetime effect on your body, mood, and physical health. Your diet may help prevent some chronic diseases and speed up your recovery time after accidents. We will go over how you can change your lifestyle, what you should eat, and other ways to get the maximum benefits of juicing. Bad gut health has been shown to influence your moods, your energy level, and how you feel in general. This book will cover the benefits of using celery juice to detox, improve your gut health, and have more energy.

Juicing can change your life as it has changed many others. You will learn about the myths and misconceptions about celery juice. We will work together to change the way you think about juicing and food nutrition. You may be asking yourself, why drink celery juice instead of just eating it? Juicing provides all the benefits of eating celery and more. It separates the juice from the ribs in the stalk that tend to get stuck in your teeth and cause annoyance. In addition to separating the ribs from the stem, it is easier to digest and detoxify your body. We will also cover seven steps to help make juicing part of your daily life and exactly what a juice cleanse is. I look forward to helping you change your life with juicing like it has many others.

There are plenty of books on this subject on the market, thanks again for choosing this one! Every effort was made to ensure it is full of as much useful information as possible. Please enjoy! Now let's head to the store!

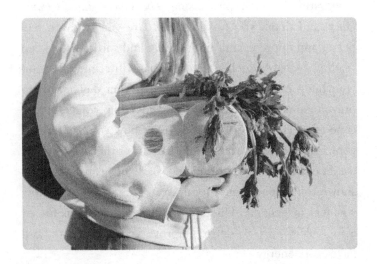

What Is the Celery Juice Cleanse?

WHY CELERY JUICE CLEANSING IS SO POPULAR

A juice cleanse is a healthy way to detox your body. The way juicing works is using a juicer to squeeze the fresh juice from the fruit or vegetable, separating the liquid from the pulp. Fruits and Vegetables are essential to your health. Fruits are high in vitamins, minerals and are anti-inflammatory. Trying to make sure you eat the right amount of vegetables day to day can be a difficult, if not impossible, task. When juicing is part of your daily life, you get all of the vitamins and minerals in one drink.

Americans are always in a hurry. Most of the time, it's easier to stop at Mcdonald's to grab a breakfast sandwich on your way to work. After a full day at work and the errands after work, it is easier to grab a pizza for dinner. Another thing many of us enjoy doing is having a nice relaxing dinner eating out. It solves the hassle of cleaning up after eating and allows you to have a much-needed break. When we aren't grabbing take-out or eating out, Our dinner may consist of boxed or frozen dinners filled with additives, high sodium, added sugars, and fat. These dinners don't taste as good as fresh food, and they make our liver work harder to break the food down. Juicing helps the liver to detox and recover from this type of diet. Foods that are high in fat or loaded with chemicals slow down your liver's ability to break down foods as efficiently as it needs to. A juice cleanse can help your liver have time to detox and rest so that it can work its best.

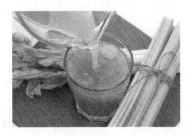

Your gut has such an influence on your body, from your mood to your day-to-day energy. Everything you eat is broken down in there. Digestive systems contain healthy bacteria and immune cells that help to fight off infections and viruses. Another job of the intestines is to communicate with the brain. The brain is what decreases the risks of depression and gives you energy. Giving your gut time to detox and rest is an essential part of your overall health.

The liver's primary function is to filter the blood from the digestive tract before it goes to the rest of your body. Your liver also filters and detoxifies chemicals and drugs. The drugs that it detoxifies can be prescription, illegal, or vitamins, and your liver does not know the difference. A juice cleanse gives you the vitamins and minerals you need therefore lowering the number of vitamins you take. The anti-inflammatory properties found in celery juice may limit the amount of medication you take to get the same benefits.

When you eat, your liver has to break down the food to get the nutrients. Your body then sends the nutrients to all the cells to energize your body. When you are juicing, it extracts those vitamins, so your body doesn't have to. Doing this gives you more energy.

If your goal is to lose weight juicing can help with that. The juice helps you feel full for a more extended amount of time, therefore, decreasing the amount of food you consume. The toxins being flushed from your body also aids in weight loss. Some of the weight loss, in the beginning, will come from water weight, but in changing the way you eat and your relationship with food, you will lose fat instead of water weight. One key in juicing is changing the way you eat. While juicing, you consume less fat, decreasing your cholesterol and therefore decreasing your heart disease or stroke risk.

Juicing also helps your skin look fresher and clearer. Your body no longer has to break down all of your food. Instead, the juice goes straight to your cells. You will look healthier, feel better, and get a glow that wasn't there before. Juicing is excellent when you are sick; it breaks down the juice for you. It keeps your immune system healthy to prevent sickness. A healthy immune system can also help with chronic conditions like allergies.

Juicing can also help you sleep better. Eliminating coffee and alcohol from your diet enables you to go to sleep more comfortably and sleep longer. Juicing increases your fiber intake, which is one of the keys to better sleep.

You haven't been eating junk food all day, and this helps your sleep cycle improve. After reading so much about the celery juice cleanse and how it has helped countless people feel better and increase their energy, you may want to give it a try but wonder where to start. It's a straightforward program. Just start adding it to your morning routine— each morning, when you get up, drink a glass of celery juice. Typically you should drink 16oz, but you can start with less and work your way up.

The first and most important thing is to drink the juice every morning for a month. Drinking it daily helps you get the maximum benefits and gives you time to see how you feel. Another thing you must remember it does not add anything to your juice. In order to get the full benefits, the juice needs to be free of any additives. Daily, people are coming up with ideas to add this or that to the juice cleanse, but that will defeat the purpose of giving your liver a chance to reset. Even if you add protein powder, thinking it will help, it will dilute the juice. Some people who start this cleanse wonder what is the difference if I throw the celery in with my morning smoothie? There is a big difference. Juicing is when you extract the water and nutrients from the fruits or vegetables, and smoothies blend the whole fruit and vegetable skin. The fiber that is in the stalk needs to be removed to get the benefits of celery.

What do you do in the morning when you get up? Do you, like so many, start brewing coffee or drink a glass of water first? The good news is you can keep that glass of water then wait 20 minutes or so to drink your celery juice. While you wait, you can start juicing the celery. In about as much time as it takes to start your coffee, you can have the juice ready.

Once you drink the juice, you need to wait another 20-30 minutes to eat breakfast. Eat something simple, a smoothie, some fruit, or oatmeal. It is vital to make the oatmeal with water and not milk. One of your goals with the celery cleanse is to detox your liver. Staying away from fats is essential while you are doing the cleanse.

If you eat fats while doing the juice cleanse, it causes the liver to break down the food instead of giving it time to heal. Not only does eating foods high in fat cause your liver to start working it will also dilute the celery juice. Diluting the juice is something you want to avoid. We want your liver to relax for a month and let the celery juice do its job. Some examples of the fats to avoid are Avocados, all dairy, eggs, and cooking oils. The good news about this is you can eat healthy carbs.

When you think of the celery juice cleanse, you probably think of Anthony William (the Medical Medium). The Medical Medium published a book in 2015 about celery juice's celery juice's healing benefits ad caught on like wildfire. Many people have become a fan of him due to his holistic approach. If you look on Instagram, you will notice he has 1.6 million loyal followers.

On Instagram, look at the Medical Mediums before and after pictures of what celery juice has done for people. It's no wonder this detox has caught on. From clearer skin to a healthier digestive tract, it appears that a lot of people have a positive experience in using the juice and what it does for them. Word of mouth is one of the best ways to tell people about a new product working for you, and this also helped celery juice gain its popularity.

Markets started to see the sales of celery going up, at times making it difficult to keep it in stock. Markets also see an increase in sales whenever medical reports indicate a product has health benefits or a celebrity or scientific claim. Now, if you search online for celery juice, you will see over 56 million results.

To further increase its popularity, celebrities' such as Sylvester Stallone, Liv Tyler, and Gwyneth Paltrow say how much the celery juice has benefited them. Stars are looked up to, and once they endorse something, others are bound to try it. Juicing continues to gain popularity as more people try it and share all the benefits. Today, many say the celery juice diet craze is a global movement and believes it is here to stay.

In an interview with the Washington Magazine, Gwyneth Paltrow said she does not need to cleanse at all. In the article, Paltrow also adds, the only time she does a cleanse is if she's doing it for her website; otherwise, only a yearly cleanse. Surprisingly, an article in her magazine, Goop, written in 2016, about the benefits Anthony Williams is said to be one of the most unconventional yet insightful healers today.

The Benefits of Celery Juice

THE REASON THIS CLEANSE MUST BE A
MAINSTAY IN YOUR DIET

Celery has not been studied as much as other vegetables, so we are just discovering the benefits of this vegetable. Most people do not know there is a difference between celery and celery juice. At the same time, both have health benefits; they are not all of the same benefits. Celery stalks have fiber, where celery juice does not. During the juicing process, the celery is pressed instead of chopped so that you get pure juice.

While celery and celery juice have similar benefits juicing gives you benefits that eating it whole does not. When you juice the celery, it removes the pulp and cuts out fiber. In removing the fiber, your body can break it down and digest it. Without the liver has to work to break it down, it can detox.

I realize that we talk a lot about how amazing celery juice benefits your liver, and there is much more to learn about that hard-working organ. Juicing has numerous healing effects on your liver due to all the nutrients and antioxidants. When your liver becomes bogged down with many fats and foods filled with chemicals and hard metals, it causes it to be sluggish and unable to filter as usual.

While reading this, you will read a lot about the Epstein-Barr virus (EBV). I want to give you a bit of information about this virus to know what it means when you hear it. EBV is a member of the herpes virus family, and this is one of the most common human viruses in the world. Most people will get some form of this at some point in their lives. One way to prevent this is drinking plenty of fluids to stay hydrated and get plenty of rest. You will read many ways that celery juice helps both of these. Celery juice is very hydrating and helps you go to sleep and stay asleep longer.

The endocrine system consists of glands that produce and secrete hormones vital for many of our bodies' functions. Some of the tasks that the endocrine system supports are respiration, metabolism, reproduction, sensory perception, movement, sexual development, and growth. An underactive endocrine system's symptoms include fatigue, depression, anxiety, craziness, weight gain, hair loss, and infertility. Hormones can overproduce or under-produce; both of these are harmful to our bodies.

Juicing offers support to the endocrine system by the easily digestible nutrients that are in a concentrated form. Increasing juicing helps improve fertility and ease the symptoms of premenstrual syndrome. I'm going to mention the liver again. It is also responsible for helping to regulate and breaking down hormones and eliminating them. Celery helps to support the liver so it can bind and excrete hormones to keep balance.

This herb contains plant hormones that help to rejuvenate the endocrine system. Your thyroid is part of the endocrine system, and as we age, it gets a bit bogged down at doing its job. Celery juice helps to kick start the thyroid and bring it back to working as it should. The endocrine system helps heal many autoimmune disorders, and celery juice helps reset the endocrine system to fight against the pathogen's attack.

Sodium cluster salts, unlike table salt, this type of salt benefits your body. The cluster salts remove the toxic salts that you have been adding to your food for years. When you have blood tests done, they may pick up the added sodium. The tests do not know the difference between healthy and unhealthy sodium. It is also possible to pick up the sodium that breaks down in your body due to the flush.

During a celery juice cleanse, you are replacing high sugar drinks with healthier options. It's interesting to note that drinks like soda, coffee, energy drinks, and specialty coffees increase our sugar intake by 50% and add 500 extra calories. Celery is antioxidant-rich. It has been shown that eating food high in antioxidants can lower the risk of chronic ailments, such as heart disease and diabetes.

Drinking as little as 250mg of celery juice three times a day is enough to keep your blood sugar at an average level. For people who have diabetes, built-up fat causes a lot of inflammation in the body that can cause kidney complications; celery juice reduces inflammation. Celery's antioxidants properties can help to reduce inflammation. While celery juice might not cure diabetes, it can help keep your blood sugar under control and help relieve symptoms. Another interesting fact is that in September 2015, a study conducted showed that the flavonoid luteolin, a nutrient in celery, might help in diabetic neuropathy or nerve damage.

Some have said that drinking celery juice every day has helped them recover from addictions. One of the causes of addiction is EBV, which is caused by the build-up of hard metals in your body. When you go through detox, your body dehydrates. Celery is made of water and keeps you hydrated. Our brain and liver go through a lot of damage during drug or alcohol addiction. Celery juice helps to reverse that due to the healing properties contained in the juice. Experts believe that many addicts are insulin resistant. Celery has a very low glycemic index which helps to even out blood sugar.

Strep, sinusitis, and strep are common symptoms of EBV in early life; this could contribute to acne. Typically, you will be prescribed antibiotics to help fight the infection when you have one of these illnesses. Medical research and science are under the misconception that acne is due to hormones. The excess oils found on skin that's thought to cause acne are sebum oil trying to fight the strep bacteria. The clusters of sodium salts found in celery help break up the strep, while the vitamin C in the juice clears up the acne.

I don't know if you have ever had to deal with a sinus infection, but they are awful. Your ears hurt, your nose hurts, your face hurts, your whole body hurts from sinuses. Some people who have chronic sinusitis opt for surgery to see if it can fix the problem. The surgery does help for a short time, and then they come back, and it can be worse than before. Drinking celery juice long-term can help with sinus issues. The sinuses are ties to the lymphatic system, and celery juice quickly reaches the sinus cavity and boosts the body's immune system.

Arthritis is a painful and chronic disorder that is caused by inflammation in one or more joints. There are multiple types of arthritis-like RA (Rheumatoid Arthritis), PsA (Psoriatic Arthritis), and Scleroderma. Each of these is believed to be an autoimmune disorder when there are indications that it may be part of the Epstein-Barr Virus. The Epstein-Barr Virus causes inflammation in joints and nerves. We already know that celery juice is full of anti-inflammatory properties, so drinking it makes sense.

The liver is one of the only organs of the body that can heal itself. When it gets overrun with toxins, you will notice you become sluggish, and so your digestive system does too. When it stops functioning correctly, your kidneys and skin have to work harder. This more challenging work causes your skin to hold more impurities that the liver usually eliminates. Celery juice helps break down these toxins so that your liver can work more effectively, which helps to clear up your skin.

In America, 6 in 10 adults have a chronic disease, and 4 in 10 have two or more. Tobacco use, poor nutrition, lack of physical activity, and excessive alcohol use are the main risk factors of chronic diseases. Celery juice has been shown to reverse some of these effects on your body. Drinking celery juice each day helps the cravings of eating foods high in sugar, and instead, you are drinking juice full of unique nutrients. The hydration and healing benefits help with the hydration and healing of your body.

Celery juice increases bile strength as a part of the

process of healing the liver. Most people are not fond of the increased bile, but it fades as the liver heals. It is excellent for people who have had their gallbladder removed by helping the liver recover. Once your gallbladder is removed, it becomes more difficult to digest substances in many foods we eat daily. A robust, healthy liver is essential in helping to break down and digest these substances.

Fibromyalgia is a chronic pain syndrome caused by the brain and nerves overreacting to pain signals. The effects of it on an individual differ from person to person, the symptoms are varied, and it can take years for a diagnosis to be made. While there is no cure for fibromyalgia, there are ways to control it, many of these consist of different types of medications and a healthy diet. Celery juice is wonderful to incorporate as part of your diet, especially with its anti-inflammatory properties. While it will not help you, it may help you to get over the inflammations quicker.

This miracle juice can also help with respiratory issues like asthma and bronchitis. Determining what your asthma trigger is essential in determining the best way to handle it. Do you frequently forget your inhaler or have to search endlessly for it? If you are going on an outing with friends or family, will there be something in the air that will affect your asthma? These are typical questions that people dealing with chronic disorders need to ask themself.

There are different types of asthma, and some of them have underlying vital conditions. Epstein-Barr is a common virus that is the reason for many chronic disorders that the medical community has not been studied. Another cause could be the toxic and heavy metals that we are exposed to daily. Emotions, stress, and mood disorders can mimic the symptoms of asthma. Think about if you have ever had a panic attack. What were your symptoms? I bet there was difficulty breathing, feeling a heavy pressure on your chest, and sometimes hyperventilating like it was almost impossible to catch your breath. There are many instances where people went to the hospital thinking they were having an asthma attack or even some who believed they had a heart attack. It is easy to see why asthma can be confused by other issues that many of us suffer.

Now let's talk about mucus, its function, and how it relates to our respiratory system. Mucus is a much-needed substance. It is a protective substance that is used in a variety of areas of our body. A major component of mucus is mucin. It is located as a lubricant, barrier, or dense material, which means that mucus protects our body's surface and assists our immune systems.

What happens is when the mucus starts fighting off infection, it can trap bacteria which causes phlegm. The phlegm is responsible for respiratory issues. Asthma, bacterial and viral infections cause your airways to make too much mucus, and This is where celery juice can help. Hydration is an essential part of thinning the mucus, so it is easier to remove it from your system. We already know that celery juice has excellent detox properties that will remove the toxins and heavy metals in your body.

Unlike many herbs, there isn't a limit on how much celery you can consume. You can safely drink multiple glasses of it without the harmful side effects. It is also interesting to note the essential oil in celery juice helps with anxiety and gout. Celery can also be used as a relaxant which is a great way to relieve pressure. Gout is caused by the buildup of uric acid in the body. Celery has compounds that break up the uric acid helping the inflammation to recede and

Most of us have heard of the mid-afternoon crash when all of our energy seems to fade, and all we want is a nap or a sugary treat. Celery juice helps to keep that mid-afternoon tiredness away. With many foods, drinks, and sugary foods, a sugar spike comes after eating them, and it fades away after a short time. The benefit of celery juice is there is no spike in energy; it is a steady stream that lasts all day.

After the 30 day cleanse, should you keep drinking it? Many people do stop drinking it every morning but continue drinking it 2-3 times weekly. They want to keep the health benefits they noticed during the 30 day cleanse. Yes, the taste takes a bit of getting used to, but you start looking forward to it once you get used to it.

In continuing to make celery juice part of your daily ritual, you keep getting the day-to-day benefits, keep your gut and digestive system healthy, detox your liver and keep eliminating unhealthy heavy chemicals you ingest. Getting celery in your diet means you will get a ton of nutrients in your diet also. You will continue to keep hydrated, and replacing those high sugar drinks is not suitable for your health.

Celery helps to support digestion. Often known as the natural laxative, celery also works as a natural way to balance your pH. You don't need a lot of these enzymes to build up weakened digestive walls. In balancing the pH, it can reverse many digestive issues such as bloating, constipation, and many other stomach issues. If your stomach acids are low, this decreases your energy levels while your stomach is digesting food. If you frequently get ulcers or have acid reflux, celery increases your gastric mucus.

Other than your overall health, one of the best benefits of celery juice is the increased energy. It is a great way to wake up with energy and a good mood before a long day. There is no caffeine in the juice, so you do not have to worry about continuously drinking highly caffeinated drinks. The beta-carotene in celery juice is converted to vitamin A, which protects from cell damage, providing you with increased daily energy.

While drinking celery juice every day, even with the many benefits, is not a magic cure-all. Suppose you continue to eat unhealthy foods and continue with a high-stress life while not benefitting as much. Without combining celery juice with a healthy lifestyle, your body will have to work too hard to get all of the benefits. If you do not enjoy its taste and can't do it daily, try to work towards doing it 1-3 times a week.

The celery juice cleanse similar to any other diet change while offering the same benefits to everyone. The cleanse will affect everyone in different ways and at different times. Someone may see the benefits the next day and another person in a week. A person's eating style will have an impact on how their system detoxes. The person who does not eat much meat and instead fills up on vegetables will likely have an easier time detoxing than the person whose primary diet consists of meats, potatoes, and desserts.

Notable Toxins to Be Aware Of

FROM ALERGIES TO PESTICIDES

❦

W hen people hear about something new, something that sounds too good to be true, people are understandably skeptical. Due to the lack of scientific studies on celery, there is a lot unknown about the benefits. There are many rumors and untruths out there about celery juice. In this chapter, we are going through some of the most frequent rumors and giving you the correct information. Celery is a unique Vegetable filled with so many vitamins, minerals, and healing abilities. Instead of doubtful, I want to ensure you know the full benefits of drinking it with confidence.

MANY SAY DRINKING CELERY JUICE IS A FAD AND WILL fade away like so many trends do. One is the amount of detox cleanses that have claimed to work wonders for your body. It makes sense that people would believe this is a fad based on the information alone. The celery juice cleanse is different because other detoxes want you to stop eating while doing the detox. We don't want you to stop eating, just make better nutritional choices and steer clear of fats.

Toxins

There are natural toxins in every food you eat. The difference between natural toxins and harmful ones is they are natural and do not contain enough toxins to cause damage. Toxins that naturally occur in fruits and vegetables are beneficial to your health. Pink rot occasionally happens in a fungus that occurs when the celery is wilting and going bad. This fungus rarely occurs and is not toxic to humans. Still, it does lower the benefits of celery juice.

Food allergen

SOME PEOPLE MAY BE ALLERGIC TO CELERY, HOWEVER very few people are allergic to celery juice. Many times what people are experiencing is the effects of the celery juice clearing out the pathogens, killing the viral bacteria are destroyed, and this releases whatever was fueling the harmful bacteria. The neurotoxins and viral waste will be going into your bloodstream for elimination which can cause the feeling of food allergies. If the celery juice triggers an instant allergic reaction, it would be because the juice instantly expelled the toxins out of our liver, or it could come from an instant shock to our system. If this is the case, change to cucumber juice and slowly incorporate the celery juice into the cucumber juice until your body can handle the full celery juice. If it is an actual allergy, please discontinue using celery juice and switch to cucumber juice or another juice that will work for you.

Psoralens

THIS IS A COMPOUND FOUND IN ALL FRUITS AND vegetables, and while people say they make your skin sensitive to light, there is no scientific or medical proof. Many medications people take have the warning that they can make them susceptible to the sun. Psoralen is good for you and is what helps to treat skin issues such as eczema and psoriasis.

Pesticides

INORGANIC CELERY MAKES THE LIST OF TOP TEN vegetables with the most residual pesticides. One way to prevent getting celery that is not full of residual pesticides you can purchase organic celery. If you can not find organic celery, you can get pesticides off your celery here in a few ways.

1. Wash it in saltwater - soaking celery in a 10% salt water solution for 20 minutes will get rid of most of the pesticides
2. Soaking it in vinegar will also remove leftover residue from the Celery. You want to use four parts water to 1 part vinegar for 20 minutes. Or

you can use full-strength vinegar - whichever one you prefer will work well

3. Clean it with baking soda and water - 1oz baking soda to 100oz of water. Soak for 12-15 minutes.

4. Just rinse it in cold water; this can reduce a lot of the pesticide

Salt content

30MG OF SODIUM IN 1 MEDIUM STALK - MAY INCREASE blood pressure and cause fluid retention. We talked about this previously in the book sodium in celery is not the same as the sodium found in sea salt or even table salt. The sodium found in celery is salt clusters that break apart the harmful salt found in packaged food and organic foods.

Oxalates

THIS MOLECULE IS TERRIBLE FOR YOUR HEALTH - oxalates are a naturally occurring molecule found in most plants and humans. Too much of this can lead to kidney stones. In plants oxalate helps to get rid of extra calcium by binding to it. Oxalates can be unhealthy if you consume too much of them like most healthy things can be harmful when done to excess.

Sugar

There is sugar in celery juice. Not all sugars are the same. Almost everything you eat has natural or refined sugars. Celery has a very low sugar content. An 8oz glass of celery juice only contains 5 grams of raw sugar. Unlike sodas and other sugar-filled drinks, it is a healthier choice. One of the main differences between natural sugars and added sugars is that natural sugar occurs naturally in foods with health benefits. Added sugars are added during the processing of packaged food and do not provide any health benefits.

Goitrogens

Goitrogens are compounds that are made of sugar and sulfate. These compounds can have undesirable effects on the thyroid and inhibit its iodine uptake. The adverse effects are an unfounded fear and have been significantly exaggerated. - while this compound is found in many vegetables, herbs, and fruits, celery is not. In reading further about Goitrogens, you will find out that it only accounts for 4% of goiter incidences or thyroid issues of the world's population.

Coumarins

Coumarins in celery are toxic to the body - coumarin is a compound found in a variety of foods. It has a sweet fragrant smell and flavor. It is also an ingredient in anticoagulant medications that promote blood circulation, preventing blood clots in your body. There is no way to know just how much coumarin is in any fruit or vegetable. It varies from field to field, state to state, and different areas of the world—the health benefits. Everything in celery juice acts together to offer immune support.

WITH ALL THE RUMORS AND CONFUSION ABOUT CELERY juice, it is easy to understand why you wouldn't know what to believe. There is so much limited knowledge it's hard to know the facts of what celery juice does and doesn't do. In the next chapter, I have made a list of the most common misconceptions to provide you with the facts instead of rumors.

Busting Myths and Misconceptions

DISPELLING COMMON MYTHS

✾

Celery juice doesn't detox your body, the detoxification process starts with the first drink of celery juice. The antioxidants that kill cancer cells immediately leap into action. It heads to your gut, working to restore hydrochloric acid, which aids in digestion; it raises the healthy stomach acid needed to break down foods and proteins. The unique compounds start working to help lower your cholesterol levels. The natural anti-inflammatory polyacetylene starts reducing chronic joint pain, gout, and arthritis. Then it starts working, helping to lower your blood pressure. Two of the most critical detoxification processes are getting the fat deposits, chemicals, and toxins out by producing health enzymes. The enzymes help digestion by flushing toxins out of your digestive tract, which increases circulation in the intestines, which helps with constipation, bloating, puffiness, and gas. This is how celery juice detoxes your body.

The Diuretic effect

DIURETICS ARE MEDICATIONS USED AS A WAY TO TREAT high blood pressure or excess water retention. Celery has a trace amount of diuretic in it. One of the benefits of celery juice is to flush out toxins. Sodium salt clusters bind with trace minerals cause the toxins to be flushed out through urination and bowel movements. While researching herb and plant diuretics, I found three of the most common ones: hawthorn, green and black tea, and parsley.

Celery Stalks Health Benefits

CELERY STALKS DO HAVE A LOT OF HEALTH BENEFITS. THE most significant difference is that the juicing process removes the fiber. The removal of the fiber makes the juice easier to digest. One of the benefits of drinking celery juice is that it is anti-inflammatory. It starves off the pathogen, flushes out and breaks down viruses, balances your pH, and restores and detoxes your digestive tract. Another benefit of drinking the juice instead of eating celery is it is a good source of vitamin k, folate, and potassium. It is much easier to drink the juice instead of eating an entire bunch of celery.

You Do Not Need to Drink Celery Juice on an Empty Stomach

ONE OF THE BEST BENEFITS OF CELERY JUICE IS IT

detoxes your liver. When you drink it on an empty stomach, it allows the liver to start healing instead of breaking down a meal's carbs. If you like, you can drink water or water with lemon before having celery juice. Wait 15-20 minutes before drinking your juice.

The Juice May interact with Blood Thinners Due to Vitamin K

VITAMIN K CAN INTERACT WITH WARFARIN; IT IS recommended to take roughly the same amount daily. Like any kind of new health plan or exercise, talk to your doctor.

There is no science behind the celery juice movement

THERE IS A LOT OF SCIENCE THAT DOES NOT KNOW about celery. It has been understudied for years. Science still has not learned about the difference between table salt and the type of salt found in celery. Celery has crystallized salt that breaks down table salt and rids it from the body. They know that the vitamins and minerals in the celery juice are healthy and help to rid the body of toxins. The hydrating content helps with many digestive system issues, improves skin, and flushes the body.

Kidney Issues

CELERY JUICE IS ONE OF THE TOP TEN JUICES FOR THE bladder and kidneys. Celery is known to remove toxins and contaminants from your kidneys. Celery juice helps to protect from kidney disease. It is also high in vitamins C, B, A, and iron, which help kidney function.

Celery Juice has Nitrates and Nitrites

NITRATES AND NITRITES ARE TWO DIFFERENT TYPES OF compounds. Both of these compounds are stable and do not cause harm. There is confusion between the nitrates found as additives in food products and those that occur naturally. The ones that occur naturally, like in celery, lowers blood pressure and make exercising more effective.

Drinking Celery Juice is Not a Cure-all

NO, IT ISN'T A CURE ALL, NOTHING IS. IF YOU DO NOT eat right, sleep well, and work to have a healthy lifestyle. Juice does heal; you can't expect overnight results. Eating fresh real food and staying away from over-processed packaged foods improves the celery juices' beneficial effects.

Should I Add other Ingredients To My Juice?

ADDING OTHER FOODS, POWDERS, OR INGREDIENTS INTO THE JUICE

Adding other foods, powders, or ingredients into the juice Is not recommended. It dilutes the juice, and you take away from the benefits. The list below all have gifts, just not added with your celery juice. Celery juice, in its purest form, has the most benefits for you. Some things that people suggest adding to the juice are the opposite of what you're trying to accomplish.

Apple Cider Vinegar

While it is alright for you, if you put Apple cider vinegar it in your celery juice, it will ruin its benefits. One of the benefits of celery juice is that it breaks down the acid in your body and flushes it from your system. Adding something high in acid to your juice would defeat the purpose.

Apples

WHILE ADDING APPLES TO YOUR CELERY JUICE TO sweeten it up may sound like a good idea, but it will dilute the healing benefits. The apple will keep the salt clusters from breaking down.

Ice

ADDING ICE TO CELERY JUICE MIGHT MAKE IT COOLER and dilute the strong flavor of the juice. But it will thoroughly cut any benefits that are in the juice, and it will be useless. It's important to note that water and celery juice are very different.

Lemon Juice

WHILE LEMON JUICE IS GREAT WITH WATER, DO NOT drink it with celery juice. It dilutes the healing properties.

Fruit

YES, FRUIT IS AN ESSENTIAL PART OF YOUR DAILY DIET. Just not with your celery juice. If you want fruit, have it in your afternoon smoothie or a late-night snack, Any fruit added to celery juice will ruin the effectiveness.

Greens

SIMILAR TO ADDING VEGETABLES TO YOUR CELERY JUICE, adding greens have a similar effect. It will hinder the production of natural electrolytes that celery juice promotes. It also causes the brain to work harder to get the same benefits.

VegetableJuice

VEGETABLE JUICES ARE GREAT TO DRINK, AND JUICES ARE beneficial. Vegetable juice added to the celery juice will cause your liver to work harder, which negates a detox's purpose. If you are going to add vegetables or vegetable juices, add them to the smoothie you drink later in the day or to another juice.

Collagen

COLLAGEN HAS MANY INCREDIBLE BENEFITS; IF YOU'RE looking to tone up and feel better, this is a great addition. If you use it with your celery juice, it will put too much bacteria into your gut, causing bloating and constipation. If you are going to use collagen supplements, do not add them to your celery juice. Drinking celery juice gives you a substantial immune boost. Taking collagen powder does the same again. If you use celery juice and collagen supplements, it will overload your immune system, and too much good at one time can be unhealthy.

Protein Powder

TOO MUCH PROTEIN IS HARMFUL TO YOUR KIDNEYS. THIS does not mean that it is terrible for you. Protein helps you gain muscle when you're not overdoing it. One of celery juice's main benefits is detoxing your kidneys.

Activated Charcoal

THERE ARE MEDICAL CONDITIONS THAT CAN BE aggravated by using charcoal. Dehydration is one of the side effects and is the opposite of what you're trying to do with celery juice. It also is not suitable for those that have constipation or slow digestion. These are both conditions that celery juice improves. Why add something to your juice that does the opposite of what you are achieving.

Fiber

WHY NOT JUST EAT THE CELERY OR BLEND IT INTO A smoothie. Celery is an herb, and the juice is a tonic. Typically when using an herb, you don't use the whole thing. In removing the fiber, you are getting more of the celery's nutrients since it is easier to digest. You aren't missing the fiber from the celery when juiced. You can get it from many other foods and green leafy vegetables.

Leaving in the Pulp

IF YOU LEAVE THE PULP IN, YOU MESS THE NATURAL detoxing properties. You do not have to worry about it being too bland or think if I put this or that in it, It'll be better; That's just not the case. If you do not want to waste the pulp, there are many things you can do with it. Use it for soups; Instead of using cream of celery soup, use the pulp. Make hummus with it and enjoy the added benefits. Another good idea is to make a face mask from it. Celery is so hydrating it would make a great mask.

Using Celery Tablets and Powder

WOULD YOU EXPECT TO GET THE SAME BENEFITS FROM an orange as you would get from one ground up or make into tablets? It is the same thing with celery power and tables. Using tablets or mixing dried celery in water will not have the same healing benefits as celery juice. Why waste the extra money when you get more help from the juice.

Will my Bowel Movement be Colorful?

NO, THE ONLY CHANGE YOU MAY SEE IS A SLIGHTLY green tint, and that happens if you drink a large quantity of the juice. While you won't experience a difference in color, you will notice a change in frequency. Bowel changes are regular and part of the detox process. If you notice loose stools, it is part of the liver removing toxins and will stop in a few days. If the loose stools and frequent bowel movements are too inconvenient, drink less celery juice and work your way up to the 16oz recommended.

HPP and Bottled Celery Juice

❧❧❧

When you buy your celery from a juice bar, ask how it is prepared to make sure they are using fresh celery. Oddly enough, Some places add a drop of bleach in the water when washing the celery. That will ruin the benefits and possibly make you sick.

IF YOU ARE DRINKING YOUR JUICE FROM A BOTTLE, MAKE sure the bottle does not say HPP. HPP stands for high-pressure pasteurization, which means it has been on the shelf that day but was made and delivered by a manufacturing plant. Juices that are made at manufacturing plants are not cold-pressed or fresh. Drinking any liquid that is manufactured has been pasteurized. Pasteurization ruins the secondary compounds and limits the juice's effectiveness. Make sure you check the ingredients in the bottle. If it's pure celery juice, it shouldn't take long to read them.

Make sure the first ingredient is celery juice; if not, it doesn't have much liquid.

JUICES FROM JUICE BARS ARE SELDOM FRESHLY SQUEEZED but instead come from concentrates or prepackaged. Usually, the only fresh-squeezed juice comes from oranges. Like the bottled juices, concentrated juices have been pasteurized, have added sugar. The healthy enzymes have been destroyed. The enzymes only come from celery juice that has been freshly juiced.

ANOTHER THING TO KNOW ABOUT JUICE BARS IS THAT their juices have been sweetened with orange, carrot, beet, or apple juice added to it. If you do get your juice from a juice bar, one thing to remember is the added sugar could do more harm than good. Concentrated sugar will feed Candida and overwhelm your endocrine system. Candida is a fungal infection caused by yeast and can cause an infection.

THE BEST WAY TO DRINK CELERY JUICE IS FRESHLY MADE at your home, so you know what is in it.

The Lifestyle to Match

W hy do you want to cleanse? Do you want it to be a lifestyle or something you occasionally do?

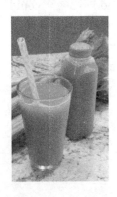

THE REASON PEOPLE START A cleanse is to reset their liver. Eating and drinking unhealthy food takes a toll on your body and leads to weight gain. A juice cleanse gives your liver and other organs a chance to flush out toxins and work more effectively. Another reason people juice is to try to change a habit. Maybe you want to start eating healthier, exchange a bag of chips for grapes. A cleanse gives your body a chance to flush out the chemicals you have been eating and start making healthier choices. One of the best ways to get the most out of drinking celery juice is to drink more water. You can drink a glass of water either before or after drinking juice. If you like the taste of lemon, add one to your water for the alkalizing effect and benefit your digestive system. It's important to remember to wait 15-20 minutes between drinking the juice and drinking the water.

Breakfast can be tricky for a few reasons. It's the first meal of the day. We're often in a rush to get out the door and want something quick. When people think of breakfast, they think of eggs, sausage, and toast; there are many other options. Swap out the breakfast filled with fat to a healthier option like oatmeal with some fruit and a morning smoothie. Some people aren't grapefruit fans, but if you are, grapefruits have significant health benefits. Just don't make the mistake of putting sugar on it. Low on time? Grab a banana, an apple or, some people make the overnight oats; these are quick breakfast options.

It's a good idea to limit the number of animal products you eat. Meat is a difficult food to digest, and our bodies need a break. As you age, animal products tend to gather into our lower stomach area, causing that dreaded pouch. During the juicing process, there will be a breakdown of fatty deposits and heavy metals. This breakdown of fat will be eliminated through sweat, urine, and stools. People who eat fewer animal products don't eat as many calories—the amount of fat in your diet decreases, resulting in weight loss.

Dairy is another food you should eat less. Dairy is difficult to digest and is one of the top foods that contribute to clogged arteries. People who are lactose intolerant are not able to fully digest the sugar in dairy. These products can cause loose stools, bloating, and gas for people who have this issue. Lactose intolerance occurs when your small intestine can not properly digest the sugar in daily products.

Eat a well-balanced diet. Most of your calories should come from fresh fruits and vegetables and limited calories from whole grains, lean protein, and nuts. A well-balanced diet is when you eat a variety of food from the food groups mentioned above. While you're juicing, it will expose you to new fruits and vegetables, and maybe you will find some you like.

The good thing with juicing is no matter what diet you are on, juicing works with it. There are many diets people are trying for optimal health. Whether your diet is filled with healthy fats, high protein, high carb, heart-healthy, or plant-based juicing is for you. All foods you eat are going to have some type of a tiring effect on your organs.

People change their diets frequently. There was a time when Slim-Fast was highly popular, then the dinners you could order from dieting companies that would deliver to your home. If you look back on previous diets, it would be interesting to read a list of their ingredients. The diets you hear a lot about now are Keto, interval fasting, and Flexi-tarian or semi-vegetarian diet, and next year there will probably be new types. With changing diets, your body gets clogged with chemicals, toxins, and heavy metals. Juicing helps to eliminate the toxins in your body while giving you essential vitamins and minerals.

To eliminate temptation while doing a juice cleanse, here are a few suggestions that may help: Make a shopping list - make a list of healthy foods that you like and add many of them. Stick to the plan. When you do not stick to the list, it is easy to look at food and say I'll only eat one. If you have a day where you eat unhealthily, don't be hard on yourself. Eating healthy is a day-by-day process that takes work to become a habit. Get support from friends. Go for a walk with a friend, join a gym, sign up for a yoga class. Suppose you have children, get them up and moving with you. Changing your lifestyle doesn't have to be work; it can be fun too.

Do not stop eating while enjoying your daily juice. Some people have the all-or-nothing approach and use juice as meal replacements. The juice is not a meal replacement. Juicing is something you are doing to ensure you're getting adequate fruits and vegetables. It also helps you get needed nutrients and eliminate buildup in your body. Juicing also adds much-needed vitamins and minerals. If you stop eating regular meals, you probably won't sustain juicing and end up binging on junk food.

If you can limit your alcohol consumption, the benefits of your juice cleanse will last longer. Alcohol is a toxin. If you drink to excess, you will be putting the toxins back into your body, causing your liver to work harder. Alcohol dehydrates the body and puts added stress on the liver to filter this out. With the liver working so hard to eliminate the bad, it's difficult to absorb the good. Alcohol slows down brain tissue growth, and some damage can not be reversed. Cutting out alcohol will make your liver healthier and reduce your chance of developing liver disease.

Limiting or stopping nicotine is essential to your health. Juicing is said to help stop the cycle of addiction. Juicing is great for your heart, lungs, liver and reverses many chronic diseases. Some juices can hope you quit smoking or at least slow down. Some people are under the false belief that smoking calms your nerves. The exact opposite is true. Nicotine can cause anxiety and can exasperate anxiety symptoms. Detoxing and working to heal your body will not have the same effects.

There's a big difference between refined sugar and natural sugar. Natural sugars that occur in fruits and vegetables are essential for good health. Refined sugars have no benefits. Refined sugar increases your risk of high cholesterol, insulin resistance, and blood sugar spikes. Sugar will lower your energy level and raise your risk of having added health concerns. Eating natural sugar has a high level of antioxidants. The nutrients in fruit and vegetables slow down the absorption of sugar.

There are some things you can do in combination with juicing to help you remove toxins. Similar to juicing, sweating is an excellent way to remove toxins from your body. Sweating helps to increase circulation in organs, tissues, and muscles. It also helps to remove excess salt from your system and can help prevent kidney stones. Alcohol and other toxins escape through your skin through sweat.

Sweating is an excellent way to remove toxins. There are many ways to sweat, not just exercise. Native American sweat lodges are not just about having a physical cleanse but a spiritual one. Emotional detoxes are as important as physical ones. There are so many stressors in this day and age: Your job, family, finances, what if your car breaks, and many more. Taking time for yourself is essential to maximize your cleanse.

A sauna is an excellent way to remove toxins from your

body. Detoxing in a sauna works hand in hand with your juice detox; they both strengthen your heart and reduce inflammation. Saunas help sore muscles and helps aches and pains. If you are just starting to work out and do yoga the sauna will be beneficial. You can either purchase one or use the one at your local gym.

The Portable Infrared sauna is another choice; You can do right from your home. An infrared sauna works differently than a typical sauna because it heats your body from the inside out. Heating from the inside out helps to accelerate the detox process. This type of sauna also helps with sore muscles, aches and pains. Like celery juice this sauna also helps to clear your skin.

A relatively new way to detox while getting emotional healing is Chromotherapy. Chromotherapy is also called color lite therapy. Color light therapy is restoring the balance of your body by applying color. These lights are located in an infrared sauna to receive the color lights' full benefits and balance your body.

Dry brushing your skin is another way to get rid of the toxins flushed from your body. Dry brushing involves a daily massage with a dry, stiff-bristled brush. It helps remove dry, flaky skin that occurs during the winter. Other benefits include: increasing circulation, detoxifying, and helping with digestion. Dry brushing is a fast and easy way to increase your juice cleanse benefits, and it doesn't take long.

Earlier I pointed out the benefits of sweating in ways other than exercise and yoga. There are benefits of both of these in addition to detoxing. Increasing flexibility, improving your strength, improved breathing and increased metabolism. There is also a way to relieve stress and help you sleep better at night. When you have had a long busy day at work, I know it's hard to make yourself work out. Even 15 minutes of brisk walking or a nightly yoga routine can help clear your mind and release more toxins through sweat.

There is no way to do all of these daily, and maybe not even weekly; it's a lengthy list. Pick a couple and do one once a day if that's all you can do. The first few that are about nutrition and lifestyle changes are difficult. Again, start slow and work your way to better health. It would be difficult to do those things cold turkey. Make a schedule. Decide the days you are going to work out, and the day you are going to be more productive, and finally, the days you're going to do self-care. On self-care days, do gentle yoga, a hot bath, or a sauna.

Clean out your cupboards and refrigerator, get rid of all of the foods that cause temptation. Replace those foods with fruits, vegetables, and other whole foods. Make sure to get enough proteins, including fish, beans, and vegetables. Proteins help to fill you up and keep you full for more extended amounts of time. Replace the countertop foods like cake and chips with oranges, apples, or grapes when you want something sweet. I keep cherry tomatoes on my counter along with apples and oranges, for when I feel like grabbing something, I can grab one of those. Stress management is a great way to cut out junk food cravings. When you feel like eating junk, do something healthy, take a walk, do some yoga, or meditate. It has been said that craving will last about 45 seconds; if you can get through that, the worst of it will subside.

Be prepared for some side effects when your body is detoxing. There are toxins in your body that you are removed during your cleanse. These are some types of common toxins that are getting eliminated: heavy metals, pesticides, plastics, industrial chemicals, and bacterial endotoxins. The toxins are removed through your urine, stools, and sweat.

Don't stop juicing if your body has some uncomfortable symptoms when you first start the cleanse. These symptoms are natural, and everyone goes through them. Some common side effects during detox are Headaches, tiredness, and irritability. While juicing is simple to follow, it is a strong medicinal process. These symptoms mean the detox is working, and your body is healing. Your body systems are in chaos while detoxing, and while it works to stabilize itself, you won't always be comfortable. At the start of the juicing process, you are not going to feel great every day. You will have good and bad days. As time goes on, you will start gaining more energy, feeling better, less anxious, and be happier.

Food cravings will happen while you are detoxing from addictive foods like chips and sugar. Include alkaline food in your diet, avoid sugar cravings at meals by eating more protein, and choosing fruits and vegetables. Avoid fried foods by replacing them with healthy alternatives like sweet potatoes, oven-baked zucchini chips, and baked asparagus fries.

While juicing is excellent for your digestive health, you can expect a change in your bowels. At first, your bowels will become more frequent with loose stools. If you were constipated before, you won't be anymore. If you are eating more vegetables than usual, you may experience more gas and bloating than usual. Here are a few more suggestions, eat bitter vegetables and herbs, magnesium supplements, daily physical activity, and eat plenty of non-starchy vegetables.

While going through these changes, do not forget to slow down, relax and reflect on the reason you're doing this. We become focused on what's around us. We forget to stop and feel what's going on in us and our bodies. Throughout your day, pause, notice what's around you, find something that makes you laugh, and always find joy in your day.

Consistency is the key to changing your lifestyle. Establish clear goals and achievable expectations. If you start something, then stop right away, then you don't get the benefits because you quit halfway. If you practice being consistent, it will improve your chances of your effort paying off. Juicing may be something that you have to work at being consistent. After doing it for a while, you will get more used to it, and it will become second nature. If you give up too soon because you don't have enough time or taste good, or for other reasons, you will not know what benefits you did not receive.

It can take anywhere from 18-254 days to start or stop a habit, knowing that helps us realize that changing our lives will take work. It's interesting to note that habit breaking and habit formation are linked in our brains; if you want to quit an unhealthy habit such as eating chips, you need to start a healthy practice like eating an apple. Your motivation matters. What is the reason you want to change the habit? If it's not a reason that is important to you, then it will not stick.

All of the suggestions listed above are just that; suggestions. They are not rules or things you must do to benefit from a cleanse. If you can't do them all, that's understandable, don't beat yourself up. If you can do a few of them, then that's great. You may also backtrack, and that's okay. You can't fail; it's a learning process and a choice.

PART I
THE SEVEN STEP CLEASING FORMULA

A Seven-Step Plan on How to Execute the
Celery Juice Cleanse

During a cleanse, you are going to need a lot of willpower. It is so easy to give in to the temptation to snack on something unhealthy. Once you give in to temptation, it may cause you to be hard on yourself, forgetting to be kind when making mistakes. Starting a juice cleanse is going to cause you stress, especially if it is something new. One way to help minimize the stress making a plan.

I have created a 7 step plan for you to help you start the juicing process and identify the benefits you want to gain from it. When you finish the day and are able to avoid temptation, allow yourself to feel proud. That is amazing you did it. Avoid high-stress situations as best you can. Some people, when stressed, tend to self-soothe with food. Having a well-developed plan will limit some stress, making the cleanse more manageable and more enjoyable.

Stress causes complications within the adrenal glands causing damaged tissues. If you are under constant stress, it triggers fight or flight responses and puts your body under strain. According to medical research, high or continuous pressure increases your chance of heart disease. Through reading this book, we have learned that juicing can reverse the effects of stress and what it does to the body.

Step 1: Decide When to Start Your Cleanse

WHY ARE YOU MAKING THE CHOICE TO CLEANSE?

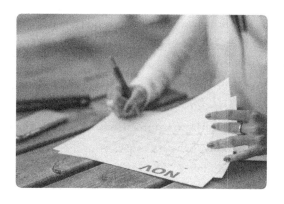

Normally, people decide to cleanse for liver health. Overeating junk keeps your body from functioning correctly and efficiently. Your body is getting to rest during a cleanse because it isn't working hard to digest foods. Is this enough of a reason for you to start drinking celery juice daily? Do you need more reasons to start the cleanse?

Do you wake up sluggish, sometimes it is almost like you woke up more tired than you felt when you went to sleep? If there is no medical reason for what you are experiencing, I will look at my daily habits. Are you working at a desk all day long without much physical activity? Are you going home, grabbing a quick unhealthy dinner, sitting on the couch watching television until you go to bed? If you answer yes to these questions, you might want to do a celery juice cleanse.

Lose some weight? If you want to lose weight, juicing is your best friend. You don't have to follow a lot of rules; there are not strict regiments. You simply add more nutrients to your body that you don't normally eat. Instead of eating at a restaurant or grabbing a burger, you can make a delicious and healthy juice. If you tend to snack during the day or while relaxing while watching TV grab some juice instead.

Do you have stomach issues? Do you suffer from a slow digestive system, do you feel sick the day after eating something unhealthy, or suffer from bloating after eating? Eating fatty foods for years causes your digestive system to become overwhelmed. The nutrients contained in juice make it easier to be absorbed. Depending on what you eat, it can take up to three hours to digest. Imagine how you and your body feels with the food setting in your stomach for that amount of time.

Step 2: Limit Caffeine

CAFFEINE IS NOT YOUR FRIEND

🙢🙠

Caffeine is not your friend. Caffeine makes it challenging to fall asleep, and sleep is vital for your body. Your body needs to rest so the juice can do its job. And caffeine increases stress hormones, and you need to avoid that during a cleanse. It causes these things by increasing your cortisol and adrenaline levels which increases energy. Caffeine slightly increases pH levels which can cause gastric ulcers, acid reflux, and irritable bowel syndrome.

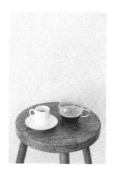

Start eliminating the primary sources of caffeine. Chocolate is a source of caffeine that many people do not realize. Energy drinks, if you think coffee has caffeine, energy drinks have so much more. Plus, energy drinks can have serious health effects, especially on children, teenagers, and young adults— caffeinated teas, like green tea and black tea. While tea has many benefits to your health, as stated earlier, caffeine has many effects that are not beneficial. Pop is loaded with caffeine, unhealthy sugars and is hard on your kidneys. Decaf coffee, while decaf coffee doesn't have as much caffeine as regular coffee, depending on where it's sourced, it may have anywhere from 0.1%-3%.

You do not have to stop caffeine suddenly; in fact, quite the opposite. I would suggest slowly cutting down. If you have ever tried quitting caffeine cold turkey, you know the severe symptoms of withdrawing. If you use multiple caffeine sources like pop and energy drinks, start sipping your pop instead of downing it. Drink half of the energy drink, half a cup of coffee. You usually want to start weaning off of caffeine the week before you begin juicing. Don't forget the water, as your body is while coming off your caffeine dependency.

A primary reason to give up caffeine during a cleanse is the purpose of cleansing is to get a break from your daily diet. Caffeine is a diuretic, and it can interfere with the natural cleanse you are trying to do while you are doing the juice cleanse. Removing toxins from caffeine causes your liver to work harder. Caffeine is one of the main things you want to avoid while cleansing.

Step 3: Eliminate Processed Food

ONE OF THE BEST THINGS YOU CAN DO FOR
YOUR HEALTH

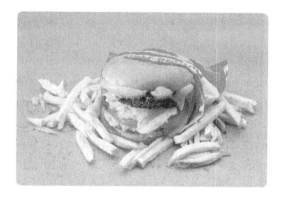

W hat are processed foods? These are foods that have been altered to be more filling, last longer, and taste better. Processed foods increase your risk of cancer because of the large amounts of chemicals in them. These foods digest quickly, meaning it does not take much energy or many calories. They contain a lot of sugar which makes sense since they're very addicting. Since they are so high in calories, it is easy to overeat them and not even realize it. Many of the ingredients in processed foods are banned in other countries because of the chemicals they contain. It's scary to think that some common foods we eat aren't even allowed in other countries because they are unhealthy.

One of the best things you can do for your health is to eliminate processed foods. You are going to start juicing. Your goals are to detox and feel great. Then you look at that box of macaroni and cheese thinking, should I? One package won't hurt, right? Yes, yes, it will. Processed food has little if no health benefits. If you look at the ingredients, there are many of them, and most you can't even pronounce.

Eliminating processed foods helps to improve your health. It improves your brain and your mood. It improves your brain health because processed foods are filled with fat, which causes memory loss and difficulty learning. Foods that are processed have also been shown to worsen symptoms of mood disorders. When you cut out those types of foods, it will also improve your looks. The inflammatory properties cause acne and aggravate skin conditions. It is not easy to cut these foods out of your diet. They are quick and easy to make and packaged in appealing bags or boxes.

Step 4: Limit fats

FATS ARE HARD FOR YOUR BODY TO BREAK DOWN

Fats are one of the most challenging foods for your liver to break down. The deposits are highly absorbable, and they grab toxins and store them in your body. Because of how absorbent they are, they act as fuel for many viruses. In juicing, it helps break down the fat for the liver and then eliminate it. Not all fat is bad, and we do need fat in our diets. Healthy fat helps us to absorb specific vitamins that are essential for health. Any fat unused by your body's cells convert into body fat.

Bloating is one symptom of eating products high in fat. The way that fat affects our brain is they get into the bloodstream, slowing down blood flow to the brain. Fats affect your cholesterol levels, causing them to 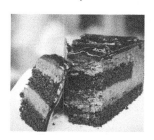 rise. It can also just make you feel gross. The juicing process eliminates the fatty deposits from your diet, decreasing your cholesterol levels, improving brain function, and helps you feel better.

Too much fat in your diet contributes to high cholesterol, increasing your risk of heart disease, strokes, and diabetes. Small amounts of fat can harm your health. A small number of fat calories can raise your risk of heart disease by 23%. Even healthy fats can cause health concerns, causing fat deposits to cause plaque to form in your arteries. Both good and bad fat can cause you to gain weight, which increases your risk of diabetes.

If you're overeating fat, it will give you bad breath, and you will need to use mouthwash and brush your teeth more often during the day. As stated many times, it will cause stomach issues, especially if you do not include many vegetables in your diet. All around, you just won't feel right. Fat causes inflammation, and that makes people feel sluggish and tired.

Step 5: Drink More Water

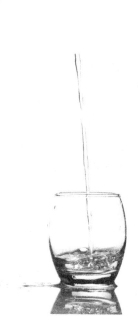

Water has many of the same benefits as doing a juice cleanse. It helps to get rid of waste through sweating, urinating, and stools. It assists the digestion process by helping your body break down food and absorb its nutrients. You can improve your mood when you stay hydrated and help your skin look healthy.

Water is an essential part of your daily life. You can't function without it. It supports the elimination of wastes and makes sure your joints have enough lubrication. It brings moisture to all tissues and organs and helps to digest food. We are continually losing water during the day through sweat, urine, and bowel movements. Juicing creates a partnership between the juice and the water causing hydration to last longer. Knowing this does not mean you do not have to slow down drinking water; just the opposite is true. The majority of your body is made up of water, making it essential to keep it working correctly.

Do you get tired during the day, drink a glass of water. Having trouble concentrating, drink a glass of water. It also helps you to control your weight because thirst can be confused with hunger. When I feel hungry at an odd time of day, I will generally drink some water, wait about 10 minutes and see if the craving goes away. If it does, I know I was thirsty and not hungry.

Experts say during a juice cleanse to drink half your weight in ounces of water. Other things that should help determine the amount of water you should consume are: Where do you live? If you live in a warm, dry state, it makes sense that you'll lose more water than someone who lives in a cooler state. What are your daily habits? Are you someone who does a lot of sitting or exercise all day? If you are an active person, you will want to drink more water.

Drinking water when you first wake up gives your organs some lubricant and helps wake up your liver. It also helps your body to flush out toxins and allows your brain to work better. If your brain doesn't get the hydration it needs, it will cause you to feel drained. If your goal is to lose weight, water will get your metabolism up and running.

You may wonder why you should juice cleanse when it seems like water does the same thing. While water does do many of the same things, there are benefits of juicing that water does not provide. Juicing helps your body to recover and detox on a larger scale quicker than drinking water. Water doesn't give you calories which could cause you to lose too many calories during the day, and you may feel drained. Juicing does provide you with calories helping to not get that drained feeling. During juicing, your immune system gets a boost with all of the additional vitamins your body is getting.

Step 6: Listen to Your Body

HOW AM I FEELING RIGHT NOW?

L earning to listen to your body may be a new experience for you. At first, it is hard to do, so often we go through life thinking we need to ignore our bodies and do what we are "supposed to." While growing up, your parents told you to clean your plate and receive a lecture if you didn't.

Some people get confused at the notion of listening to themselves. They do not realize a difference between your brain telling your body it craves something and listening to your body. How do you feel when you eat pie versus when you have an apple or salad.

When you start listening to your body, your brain may trick you. Brains learn what chemicals are released when you eat a particular food, and it wants to keep those chemicals coming. If you eat chocolate knowing that it releases serotonin which is a chemical that makes you feel good, it may help you understand why you're experiencing the craving. Knowing this may help you get through the urge, or you can see if a healthy food can cause a similar feeling.

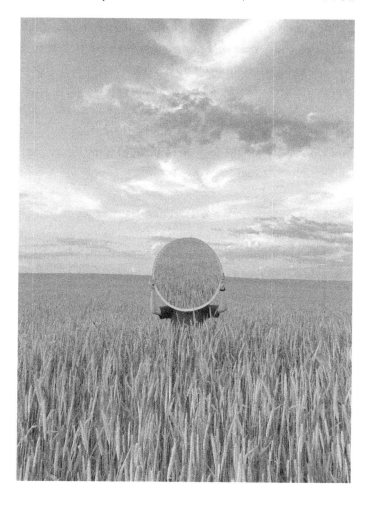

Be gentle with yourself. Learning to listen to your body isn't something that's going to come naturally. Since you were little, your parents taught you to listen to other people before yourself. There is a fear in learning to listen to yourself. As an adult if you have experienced trauma it may be hard to reconcile your thoughts, feelings and how you think you should feel or think. Listening to yourself and learning to accept yourself will probably be a long process.

Ask yourself, how am I feeling right now? If you sit quietly for a few minutes, you will probably get an answer. It won't be audible, but you will feel it. Sometimes I will ask myself if I could do anything right now, what would it be? I don't get a crazy answer like travel the world; I get a real response. One day asking myself this question, my answer was dance. I got up, put on some music, and danced, and it felt great. That is hard to remember to do.

Movement is a great way to get to know your body. Get up early, do yoga, take a walk, do something that causes you to get out of your head. Moving is a great way to connect to your body, and it brings you into the present moment. Another tool I use is meditation, one of the best ways to learn to listen to yourself.

Step 7: Choose the Correct Foods

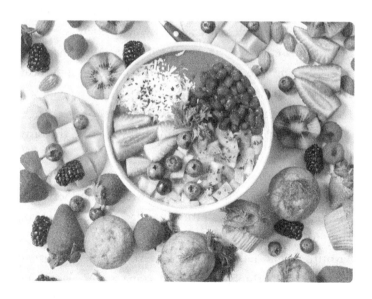

Now that you know what not to eat, let's focus on what to eat. Starting on a juice cleanse does not mean the night before you should eat a huge, sugar-filled meal willed with fats. You should do the exact opposite. Your juice cleanse will be so much more challenging if you don't prepare yourself for it by eating healthy. People will often use juicing to go back and forth between eating healthy, then going back to their old way of eating, and then starting another juice cleanse. Using cleanses and detoxes can become as addictive as using laxatives or diuretics as a way to undo the adverse effects of overeating; if you're someone that tends to do this, look into your relationship with food.

If you start changing the way you eat before starting the cleanse, you will have better results. Start eating more vegetables, fruits, nuts, and seeds, and healthy protein. Eat simple small meals that are easy to digest and are full of green leafy vegetables. If you crave soups, there are many non-creamy grain-free ones you can make. About five days after starting the juice cleanse, cravings for unhealthy foods begin to fade. Once you start eating better, you will be able to figure out when you're hungry and eat enough. You start wanting to eat healthily, and you crave the taste of fresh foods.

Add color to your plate. Not only does color make your food look more appetizing, but you will also get more vitamins and minerals. Eat a variety of salad greens. When you shop for salad greens, get a variety of greens. Look for your favorite greens and some you haven't tried before just to see what you think. There are some sweet fruits and vegetables to satisfy a craving. A few examples of sweeter vegetables are green peppers, sweet potatoes, and squash. Most importantly, don't let eating become boring, have fun, blend different flavors just to see how it tastes. If you don't already, you may just learn to love cooking.

When you start focusing on having a healthy diet, you

will start cooking at home more, eating breakfast daily, and taking your lunch to work. Since you are no longer eating processed food, you now prepare your lunch before work. Like cooking at home, bringing your lunch to work is a twofold benefit. You not only are eating better, but you're also saving money too.

Eat dinner by 7:00 pm. After dinner, you can have some raw nuts or a smoothie to help appease your hunger. Nutritionists have typically recommended having three meals a day with 2-3 snacks. Take your time while eating, make a conscious effort to pay attention to how the food tastes. It takes time for your brain to realize when you're feeling full. Never think of any food as being off-limits. When you do that, you start thinking of it more often, which may cause you to binge on them.

If you have a sluggish digestive system, you may want to start eating steamed or baked vegetables before working up to raw ones. Years of eating unhealthy foods take a toll on your digestive system. During a juice cleanse, you will be getting the enzymes you're missing, and you will notice the change in how you feel.

How to Make This a Habit that will change your life

PLAN AND EXECUTE

Juicing can be the first step in making healthier choices. When you're finished with your 30 day cleanse, you will feel amazing. You will want to continue feeling this way. Feeling good each day is possible! You can make all of the same choices and keep juicing. You have discovered many of the benefits of juicing. Why 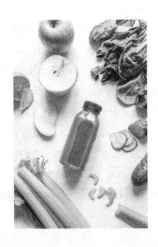 stop now. Make it a part of your daily life. Each morning make yourself a juice, just like you have been. Now, instead of just celery juice, you can start experimenting. Ask yourself the question of what benefit do you want to get from juicing. Do you want added energy? Look for a recipe that says for added energy. If you have gone to the store and read the ingredients, some combine many different juices. Seeing all the different combinations can cause you to feel overwhelmed. That's why you want to find a book or search the internet for beginner juice recipes. Beginner juice recipes will have fewer ingredients and will give you a chance to work your way up to juices with more ingredients. Beginner juicing tips can help you find the type of juicer you want or if you want a juicer. Some people use a blender and strain out the whole parts. What benefits you get from juicing are endless.

During the juice, you gave up caffeine. You've made it through the withdrawal and detox process. You can choose if you want to start consuming caffeine again or not. If you did a 30 day cleanse and gave it up for the entire time, you might want to start slowly. During this time, you have probably become more sensitive to caffeine's effects, so introduce it gradually. Don't jump right back into drinking a full cup of coffee or a glass of pop all at once. Consuming caffeine suddenly may have an adverse effect on you. If you can, try to limit the amount of alcohol you drink and don't drink any for the first week after your cleanse. Your liver enjoyed the break from working so hard let it get used to breaking down and digesting food slowly. If you can help it, do not go back to eating high sugar and processed foods. Going back to old habits will start the process of your body working hard and your liver becoming sluggish all over again.

Watch the amounts of fat and protein you're eating. When you eat fats, make sure they are healthy versus unhealthy fats. By now, you have learned the difference; use your knowledge. Make sure you're eating high-quality, skinless protein if you are eating animal products. Starting to consume dairy suddenly may have adverse effects as well.

Dairy has a tendency to cause constipation, so make sure to keep eating high fiber. While on the cleanse, you started listening to your body's needs and listening to yourself. Continuing to eat whole foods instead of junk food will help to keep you self-aware. While doing your juice cleanse, your skin started to look great. If you continue eating healthy, your skin will continue to look healthy. Be careful of sugars. It is easy for them to sneak back into your diet. Many drinks or juices that claim to be natural aren't natural. If you read the label, you may find ingredients that show their added sugars and other ingredients. Instead of drinks with added sugars, you can drink water with lemon or drink water with mint and cucumber. There are also caffeine-free and herbal fruit teas that are great options.

Don't forget to hydrate. Continue drinking enough water daily to help aid your digestion. You've been getting a lot of extra hydration during your juice cleanse, so try to decrease the hydration slowly. Continue to eat your fruits and vegetables. You have gone through the hard work of making them essential to your diet. You know firsthand the benefits. Try to aim for five servings of vegetables daily and two servings of fruit. During your cleansing, you have started exercising and exploring different ways to sweat. Keep this habit. Sweating will help you to continue to detox and flush out toxins. Keep moving! Exercising, doing yoga, walking, or stretching are all ways to continue moving. Not only does it make you healthy, but it also makes you feel great too.

Finding whole foods can be less convenient than grabbing frozen or canned foods, but the health benefits are enormous. During the cleanse, you have learned so much about the difference between whole food and processed foods. Whole Foods are full of healthy nutrients that we need to be healthy. They have raw sugar instead of processed sugar. Knowing this is important because your body is better able to process natural sugar. Whole Foods are heart-healthy. They're packed with antioxidants and rich in nutrients. Whole Foods are high in fiber, supporting a healthy digestive system and helping you feel full longer. The higher fiber content helps to keep your gut healthy because it is rich in prebiotics.

Whole Foods do cost more, and if you do not have a lot of money, this can make it hard. Do the best you can. Any improvement is a win. It can make preparing food time-consuming because you will need to plan and prepare your meals. It can lead to stress if you feel you can only eat whole foods. It is essential to remember you're doing the best you can and continue to go easy on yourself. One way to help with time is to plan and prepare your meals weekly or daily. It doesn't need to be complicated. What ingredients do you already have? Make use of the fruits and vegetables to save time having to go out shopping—layout what you will eat all week on Sunday Afternoon. Plan your meals, including snacks, and if you're going to have a healthy dessert like fruit salad, make it earlier in the week. If you don't want to do it once a week, do it for a few days in advance. Make sure the food you are preparing food you enjoy so you look forward to eating it. Enjoying what you eat is essential to your diet; if you do not want to eat your food, why bother sticking with your new plan.

If you can't or don't want to continue eating whole foods, the next best thing is learning to read food labels. Please don't believe what it says on the front of the box. Marketing companies make a lot of claims that aren't true. Always read the nutrition label and ingredient list. Always check the serving size; if a bag of frozen vegetables contains eight servings and the serving size 1/4 cup, there's a good chance it's not going to fill you up. Calories per serving are essential to read to determine your calories accurately. Check the amount of sodium that is in the food. What type of fats are in the food, no saturated fats, no hydrogenated fats. All fat can damage your heart. If you're getting grain products, make sure it is a whole grain. Reading a food label is confusing and hard to learn how to do correctly. There are so many phone apps out there now that you can probably find one that can help out.

Continue to journal. Food journaling is excellent for mindful eating. You will be keeping track of what you eat and the number of calories you are getting. Many times by the end of the day, you have forgotten what you ate earlier in the day. Journaling is a way to prevent this from happening. It also helps you to know the times of day you get the most hungry. You will discover if you are eating out of boredom or if you are an emotional eater. If you are eating out of boredom, you can find ways to distract yourself and do something healthy. Go for a walk, listen to music or get up and move. If you're an emotional eater, you can take steps to learn your triggers. If stress is a trigger, find what helps you to release tension. If being upset is a trigger for you finding ways you can find a way to feel better than with food. Learning to soothe yourself is a tool that is always needed.

Some people feel better after a nice warm bath, doing yoga, exercising, or painting. Find what works for you. You can Keep your journaling short. It doesn't have to be pages. A helpful benefit about journaling is you will find out if you have a food sensitivity and what food makes you feel better or bothers you. Food journaling can help you find out how you are eating, affecting what and how you eat. You will learn your real eating habits. Are you eating as much healthy food as you think you are? Are you trying to trick yourself into believing you are doing better than you are? These are some of the answers you will find when you keep a journal.

Afterword

Thank you for making it through to the end of *The Celery Juice Cleanse Hack*, let's hope it was informative and able to provide you with all of the tools you need to achieve your goals whatever they may be.

There is so much confusion over what the celery juice cleanse is that it's hard to decide fact from fiction. You will find out what a juice cleanse is and how it will benefit you and your body. Your body and mind are connected to the food you eat, and juicing can improve both. When your digestive system is not functioning well, you don't feel well, and it will have a negative impact on your moods. Celery juice is a great way to detox your body from all of the chemicals you consume in your daily life. If this is your first cleanse, you will learn what to expect when you begin juicing: what you should add, if anything, to your juice. You will learn about detox symptoms, how to make them less harsh, and the best ways to deal with them. A step-by-step guide will help you move through the juicing process with ease and prepare for the cleanse. You will discover if juicing is part of a lifestyle you want to keep or if you're going to use it as the occasional pick-me-up. If you're going to make it part of your lifestyle, there are suggestions on how you can do that. We will explore common myths and misconceptions about what exactly celery does and does not do. How you can incorporate juicing in your daily life and why you would want to. By the end of the book, we will help you answer whether celery juice has the benefits people claim.

Made in the USA
Monee, IL
03 November 2023

45749989R00049